HOW TO SLEEP

A Natural Method

LUCINDA FORD

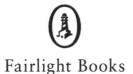

Fairlight Books

First published by Fairlight Books 2020

Fairlight Books
Summertown Pavilion, 18 - 24 Middle Way, Oxford, OX2 7LG

A CIP catalogue record for this book is available from the British Library

ISBN 978-1-912054-23-7

www.fairlightbooks.com
Printed and bound in Great Britain by TJ International Ltd
Cover designed by Amanda Weiss

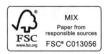

CONTENTS

INTRODUCTION

Many people, at different times in their lives, suffer from a difficulty in falling asleep. Sometimes there is a physical or physiological cause, such as acute pain, pregnancy, or the hot flushes of menopause. Sometimes it is the result of an anxious, stressed or overactive mind. It may also begin with a physiological cause, but then continue after that trigger is no longer present – the fear of insomnia proving a worry in its own right.

When sleeplessness becomes a regular occurrence, it can set up a vicious cycle: fatigue reducing your ability to cope with daily life, which in turn leads to sleepless nights. Finding ways to turn off the racing mind, the negative thoughts, the sadness or anxiety when retiring to sleep is an essential step, allowing you to break that vicious cycle and move towards a place of better well-being.

This book offers eight simple techniques designed to calm the mind and allow sleep to come naturally. They are distilled from the thinking of cognitive behavioural therapy, mindfulness and meditation, taking lessons from each of these methods on how best to quiet your mind and find a calm place from which to fall asleep.

How to use the techniques

The sleep techniques given in this book are based on three principles:

1. Relaxation and visualisation techniques can allow you to switch from an active mode to one in which sleep can naturally take hold.

2. A practice of mindfulness can help where sleep is being held at bay by an anxious or racing mind.

3. An understanding of the practices of cognitive behavioural therapy can help if sleep is being held back by negative thoughts arising uncalled for in the mind, or where internal battles are raging.

It is not essential to read the whole of this book before trying out the techniques – you can just open it at any technique and jump right in.

First, while in bed, read through the technique that you would like to try. Then turn off the light and follow the instructions for the technique, slowly, steadily, and methodically.

The aim is not to reach the end of the technique, but to allow yourself to fall asleep while you are working your way through it.

CHAPTER ONE

Establishing Why You Can't Sleep

When you think about it, the process of falling asleep is quite a wondrous thing. You close your eyes and send a signal to your body that it is time for sleep. You're not closing your eyes because they're gritty or it's too bright. You're not closing them because there's something unpleasant in front of you that you don't want to see. You're closing them because you wish to switch from the state of being awake to the state of being asleep.

Most of the things your body can do happen either because your conscious mind has willed it – 'Wiggle, toes!' your brain demands, and wiggle they do – or because another part of your brain, along with your autonomous nervous system, has taken care of it without you needing to worry. These unconscious bodily functions include your heart beating, your lungs breathing in and out, and your digestive system working away on your supper.

But falling asleep is neither quite one nor the other. You can will it, by closing your eyes, but then you have to wait for your body to agree that the time is right.

Perhaps it would be easier if the 'go to sleep' function were one of the things we could directly control, like wiggling our toes, but unfortunately, we're not made like that.

When the body is refusing to co-operate, we must find other ways to provide it with the trigger it needs to understand it is time to sleep – time to switch from 'active' mode to 'sleep' mode.

When the 'go to sleep' switch isn't working

Before introducing the first of the techniques which you can use to help your body understand it is time to sleep, it is worth spending a little time reflecting on the possible reasons why your 'go to sleep' (or your 'stay asleep') switch is malfunctioning.

For some, the cause is easily identified – I'm too uncomfortable or hot / I can't stop thinking about work / I'm feeling sad or worried about something / I'm suffering from grief – but sometimes there isn't an obvious reason, or maybe it's a complex combination of factors.

The techniques in this book are based upon several different schools of thought, encompassing both Western behavioural sciences such as cognitive behavioural therapy, and the Eastern meditative practices of mindfulness and meditation – but they all have something in common. They work to trigger your brain and body to let go of their active 'day mode' and switch on their 'sleep mode'.

Before we look in more depth at the possible triggers for why your body might be reluctant to switch into sleep mode, let's first examine how a body gets ready for action and how it subsequently gets ready to step back from action and enter into a period of rest and recuperation. Both of these things are controlled by something called the autonomous nervous system.

Thinking about your fight-or-flight response

There are functions of your body that work without you consciously making them happen – the heart beats at a regular pace, the lungs bring air in and out of your body, and the digestive and urinary systems work away to process the food and liquids you've ingested.

How does that work? Well, these unconscious functions are controlled by the body in almost the same way as our conscious actions are. The messages 'wiggle, toes' and 'beat faster, heart' are both passed from 'head office', the brain, through the nervous system to arrive at the part of the body which must act – the muscles that move the toes or pump blood through the heart, or the glands that excrete hormones to make your blood pressure rise in order to help your heart beat faster.

The only difference is that 'wiggle, toes' comes from the parts of the brain that process conscious actions, while 'beat faster, heart' comes from a very specific part of the brain called the amygdala. The amygdala controls emotional responses.

The unconsciously raised messages to your body deriving from the amygdala have their own part of the nervous system to travel through called the autonomous nervous system, and that system is made up of two distinct parts.

The first is used to get the body ready for action (for the good old-fashioned fight-or-flight response), and is called the sympathetic nervous system. It's a set of nerves that radiate from the spinal cord to different parts of your body: a system that causes your heart to beat faster, your pupils to dilate and your lungs to breathe harder and bring more oxygen to your muscles. It's geared towards making sure that you're ready to throw that punch, get those legs working to run away or generally react in the best way to protect yourself from whatever dangers are arising.

The other half of the system, the parasympathetic nervous system, looks after the day-to-day workings of the body. It supports what is commonly referred to as the 'rest-and-digest' state. In other words, the parasympathetic nervous system organises the things the body needs to do while it is in a resting or recovery phase. This includes the digestion of food and the processing of urine.

These two systems, the sympathetic and the parasympathetic nervous systems, are always at work managing your bodily functions without you having to think about it, a little like keeping a car in a steadily moving line of traffic – now a little more gas, now a little less; now a turn of the steering wheel to the right, now a quick adjustment to the left.

When something happens that needs your body to be ready to react, and which could be derived from a physical threat or an emotional one, the sympathetic nervous system dominates. When the threat has passed, the parasympathetic nervous system is allowed to step back in and get on with the day-to-day bodily functions.

What has this got to do with getting to sleep? Well, let's start off with an extreme example.

You arrive home to see a hooded mugger approaching from the darkened stairwell with a knife outstretched. A moment later, this is followed by the realisation that it's your eighty-six-year-old neighbour inviting you in for tea and a slice of her delicious homemade chocolate cake.

What's been happening to your body during this interaction? When you first felt danger was at hand, the sympathetic nervous system swung into action, activating the adrenal gland and causing it to flood the body with a hormone called epinephrine, more commonly known as adrenaline. This hormone is responsible for getting the body and its muscles ready for physical action. Next, the sympathetic nervous system caused your body to be flooded with cortisol. This makes sure the body has the energy it needs to do whatever the brain is going to decide to do (whether fight or flight) by increasing the blood pressure and releasing sugars into the bloodstream. Then the sympathetic nervous system got the heart beating faster, so as to get all that sugary blood where it needed to be, and caused the lungs to work harder to bring in more oxygen to support it all. Essentially, it got you ready to throw that punch.

Once the danger had passed, and you were sitting eating the delicious cake, laughing with your neighbour about how you mistook her for a mugger, the sympathetic nervous system stepped down. Your heart rate slowed, your blood pressure fell, and the levels of adrenaline and cortisol in your body lowered again. Finally, the parasympathetic nervous system was given its chance to step in and carry out its functions again – in this instance, digesting tea and cake.

When you thought a mugger was at hand – your face flushed, your heart pounding – it would have been difficult to fall asleep, but when your neighbour pottered off to refill the teapot, if the chair was comfy and the fire was warm, you might have been tempted to close your eyes there for a moment...

Establishing why it is hard to let go

Unlike the example given before, unless we are in a war zone or have a job which involves physical danger, our days don't usually revolve around one terrifying incident followed by a period of safe rest and recuperation. In reality, our days are often filled with a series of physical or emotional stresses, some small, some large, followed by periods of achievement, happiness or relief – again, some small, some large – constantly causing the sympathetic nervous system to kick into action and then retreat again and again.

An example day for someone might be: get up worrying about that presentation or meal that needs preparing, hurry to drop the kids off at school, be followed too closely by an inconsiderate driver, take a call from a friend or friendly colleague, laugh out loud, get to work on time for once and then find there are no parking spaces left. And it's not even 9am yet... On, off, on, off.

Someone coping with a bereavement, breakup or illness might find their day similarly filled with a mix of sadness and light relief. It's important to understand that an emotional threat to your well-being causes the same stress response in your body as a physical one. Worrying about the future, hearing someone say something hurtful about you or a loved one, receiving news of a bereavement or experiencing the daily reminder of having lost someone will all cause your body to suffer a similar physical response as thinking there is a mugger beside you. When someone says something unpleasant that makes you angry, in the same way as when your body gets ready to fight, your heart will beat faster, your muscles will tense up and your face will become flushed, because the sympathetic nervous system has leapt into action. Stress related to work, grief, depression or unhappiness all cause the same physical response in your body – which is why difficulty sleeping can be caused by any one of these things, even if you are trying to ignore them, bury them or bottle them up.

It's little wonder that when you get to bed, after your system has been constantly flooded with and then drained of cortisol and adrenaline, after the alternation of rising and lowering heart rates and of your face flushing and cooling, your body can't figure out, just because you close your eyes, that it's time to stop all that and go to sleep. Especially since, when we go to bed, a number of those threats might still be there with us – worry about a deadline, sadness about a breakup, grief, illness, concern, stress. They don't go away just because we've closed our eyes.

When you can't sleep or repeatedly wake in the night, the symptoms are remarkably similar to that of a fight-or-flight response – tossing and turning, your mind going round in circles, looking for solutions to a whole host of problems, dwelling on angry, bitter or depressing thoughts. It's as if your body has got stuck with the sympathetic nervous system in overdrive.

What is needed is for you to instruct your brain that those problems are going to be solved at a later date; they are not going to be solved when you are in bed trying to sleep. That when you close your eyes to sleep, it will be a time for rest and recuperation, a time for the body to relax and recover. That the fight can be continued at another time.

How to do that? For someone who has difficulty sleeping, being told to relax can be a red rag to a bull. They know they need to relax in order to be able to fall asleep, but they can't find a way to stop their racing mind, can't find a way to stop waking up, can't find a way to stop the negative thoughts from coming to them.

Lying in bed and willing yourself to relax can sometimes work, but as often as not it creates a new anxiety about why it's not working, causing the person to dwell on fears about the morning and how they will cope without much sleep.

Each of the eight techniques in this book, although they come from different sources and from very different ways of looking at the world (whether from a Western or an Eastern viewpoint), all share a goal of distracting your mind with another purpose and clearing it so that the body can finally switch off and relax. Often they are accompanied by practices which work against the physical effects of the sympathetic nervous system; these practices include slowing the breathing to a steady rate, relaxing the muscles and allowing the heart rate to fall. Mindfulness in particular is designed to help you keep your mind in the present moment. When you are in the present moment, it is difficult to reflect on concerns about how you will handle future battles or solve future problems, and it is impossible to dwell on past slights, to go over how you wish you had reacted or to start analysing the actions of others.

Sometimes it's hard to specifically identify how or why you are under stress, particularly if you have a habit of intellectualising your worries, putting a brave face on things or soldiering on. Sometimes it's only when you have a manifestation of your stress, sadness or anxiety, such as difficulty sleeping, that you realise the extent of the pressure you are under.

Take the questionnaire that follows and then take a few moments to reflect on the possible reasons why you may be having difficulty sleeping or may be waking in the night. There are no right or wrong answers to the questionnaire.

Sleep Questionnaire

Tick all of the answers that might apply

<u>Environmental and Physical Factors</u>

❑ The room where I sleep is not very dark.

❑ It's sometimes noisy where I try to sleep.

❑ I'm often too hot in bed.

❑ Of late, I've been drinking more alcohol than usual.

❑ I've been sleeping during the day.

❑ I've been having long lie-ins to try to catch up on my sleep.

❑ I've been going to bed earlier than I used to.

❑ I think my breathing stops and starts when I sleep.

❑ I think I make gasping, choking or snorting noises when I sleep.

❑ I sometimes have an uncontrollable urge to twitch or touch my legs at night.

Mind and Body Factors

- ❑ When I try to sleep I start to think through the problems of the day.
- ❑ When I try to sleep I start to worry about one thing or maybe a number of things.
- ❑ When I try to sleep I start to think about things that make me sad and I start to cry.
- ❑ When I try to sleep I get angry about things that are going on in my life.
- ❑ When I try to sleep I get angry with somebody specific.
- ❑ When I try to sleep my mind is racing.

Which of these applies?

- ❑ I feel under pressure at work.
- ❑ I've recently changed jobs.
- ❑ I work long hours.
- ❑ I recently suffered a bereavement.
- ❑ I recently separated from my partner.
- ❑ I'm trying to buy or sell a house.

- ❏ I'm concerned I may not be able to cope financially.
- ❏ I have fallen out with one or more relatives.
- ❏ I'm getting married.
- ❏ I am having a dispute with my neighbour.
- ❏ I've been diagnosed with a medical condition.
- ❏ I'm worried about someone close to me.
- ❏ I'm worried about money.
- ❏ I'm worried about the environment.
- ❏ I'm worried for the safety or myself or those close to me.
- ❏ I sometimes can't stop crying.
- ❏ I feel worried a lot of the time.
- ❏ I always jump to the worst possible outcome when worried about something.
- ❏ When trying to sleep I worry that if I don't sleep I will not cope tomorrow.
- ❏ If I'm not able to do all my relaxation practices before going to bed, I can't sleep.

Mitigating environmental and physical factors

Light and Noise

Nearly all animals, including humans, have an internal process that regulates (among other things) their waking and sleeping cycle over a twenty-four-hour period, called a 'circadian rhythm'. Our bodies use external clues, like seeing whether it is light or dark, to keep the twenty-four-hour clock on track and to know when it is time to sleep and when to rise.

Ensuring that the room is dark when it is time for sleep and light when it is time to get up works with our natural circadian rhythm. On the other hand, having a light room when trying to sleep confuses and interrupts our circadian rhythm. In the same way, noise around us when we are trying to sleep provides clues to the body that action is still happening, and that the body needs to be ready to react.

It is not essential to have an entirely dark or entirely quiet room to sleep, but it is important that it is not so light nor so noisy that your body is unconsciously receiving signals that it is still daytime. Light seeping between curtains from streetlights, a partner whose snoring comes in fits and spurts, and noisy neighbours are all examples of stimulants that trigger our daytime mode rather than our sleep mode.

It is worth spending a little effort and possibly some of the household budget in minimising these disruptions.

Making It 'Night-Time'

Consider replacing your curtains or blinds if they are not effectively keeping the room dark when you want to sleep. Many shops sell curtains with blackout linings which are specifically designed to help make a room dark for sleep, or you could choose a heavier set of blinds. When the sole purpose of curtains is to darken the room for sleep, it is odd to think that many ready-made versions place the look of the curtains over their ability to function. Choose a curtain that has a choice of threads at the top on which to place the hooks. Place the hooks on the row of threads that causes the top of the curtains to reach above or touch the track or curtain pole, minimising the amount of light that can seep through the gap at the top of the curtains.

If it is not possible to change the curtains, or your budget will not stretch to that, consider buying one or two eye masks. They should be of a light material. Some luxury ones made of cashmere can feel like a treat, but they don't wear as well and need delicate washing on a regular basis.

Some people find that just a light pillow or T-shirt over their eyes is enough until they fall asleep, so you may want to try this.

To block out noise, try using earplugs. Some people complain that they have tried them and they didn't work. There are lots of different styles of earplugs, and some versions might not be a great fit for some users. It is worth experimenting to find the type that suits you best. They can be very cheaply bought at a chemist or drugstore. The soft foam ones in the shape of a bullet are generally the best, and have the added advantage of being the least expensive.

Keeping to a Sleep Schedule

In the same way that light and noise disrupt your circadian rhythm, sleeping at irregular times provides confusing signals for your body. If you are not sleeping well, it can be tempting to try to catch up on your sleep with a daytime nap, by going to bed early, or by sleeping in later in the morning, but this actually works against you. Try to keep to regular times for going to bed and going to sleep.

Heat

Around 75% of postmenopausal women experience hot flushing, a sudden intense rise in body temperature, which often occurs at night when the body's oestrogen levels drop. Women can also experience this while they are perimenopausal, particularly at the stage around one to two years prior to their periods stopping, when swings in oestrogen levels can lead to hot flushes, night sweats, mood swings and, consequently, difficulty sleeping. For several decades, doctors have commonly prescribed hormone replacement treatment (HRT) to reduce these symptoms, but recent research has proven stronger links between HRT and breast cancer. A 2019 study of 108,647 postmenopausal women, published in *The Lancet*, found an increased risk of breast cancer from use of oestrogen-progestogen compounds and (though to a lesser extent) use of oestrogen-only systemic HRT. The study also proved for the first time that increased cancer risk from HRT can last up to fifteen years after the treatment is last taken.[1]

For that reason, doctors now discuss the risks and benefits of using HRT, and many women prefer not to take it and instead to try to manage living with the symptoms of the menopause.

To combat temperature swings, choose cotton sheets over synthetic, and instead of using one large duvet or comforter, consider using layers: place a cotton sheet on top of you and, over that, a light duvet or comforter which can be quickly thrown off without disturbing your sleep or leaving you to wake, shivering and uncovered, ten minutes later. Choose cotton nightwear over synthetic or wool as it is more breathable and will keep you cooler.

If you are too hot when trying to get to sleep, or if you wake with night sweats, run your shower to cold and step in for one to two seconds, then return to bed without drying yourself. It is a very effective way of staying cool for the time it takes you to fall asleep.

Sleep Apnoea

If you think that your breathing stops and starts when you sleep or that you make gasping, choking or snorting noises while sleeping, it may be that you suffer from sleep apnoea, a condition where the airwaves become obstructed during sleep. Sleep apnoea can be caused or made worse by obesity, by taking certain sleeping pills or by smoking or drinking alcohol, so if you think one of these factors could be a cause, then you could look to address that. But it can also be caused by allergies or enlarged tonsils.

You can also speak to your doctor, who can refer you to a sleep clinic to test whether and how often your breathing stops when you are sleeping. If sleep apnoea is identified as a problem, there is a device called a CPAP machine which might be able to help. This is a mask you wear over your mouth and nose, which provides air to your airways.

Restless Legs Syndrome

Restless legs syndrome, or RLS, is a specific condition in which there is an overwhelming urge to move or twitch the legs. For sufferers of this condition, the urge can come in the evening when starting to relax or when lying in bed to sleep. According to the charity RLS-UK, it can affect 7.2% of the population at some time in their life and can lead to sleep difficulty.

It is believed to be caused by a fall in the body's levels of dopamine, a hormone produced by the brain which helps it to co-ordinate movement. A fall in dopamine can be triggered by iron deficiency anaemia. It can also be a side effect of some long-term medical conditions, and there are some medications which can worsen the effects of RLS.

If you are suffering from RLS, it is a good idea to seek advice from your doctor, who can test whether there is a medical problem causing the symptoms.

You might also want to think through whether there are any new stimulants you are taking before bed, such as alcohol, coffee or tea, remembering that herbal teas are not all necessarily calming and in fact some can be stimulating.

Sleep Rituals

If you are feeling stressed from a challenging day, it makes sense to try to create a separation between daytime and night-time. Having a relaxing bath and taking a break between reading work emails and sleep time are good for this and are often recommended as ways to help you ensure a better night's sleep. However, it is important that the preparations for sleep don't themselves become something that you feel *must* be done before you can go to sleep.

Sometimes people get into a habit of rising when they can't sleep, or of turning the radio on. Like going to bed too early or sleeping in, these habits confuse your circadian rhythm and are likely to cause you to have future episodes of waking in the night. If you can, it is better to try to remain in bed, and accept that you may be awake, but at least your body is getting rest which it wouldn't be getting if you were up and moving about. If you wake in the night, try using one of the techniques in this book to get back to sleep again.

If you think you might have developed rituals for getting to sleep or for when you wake in the night which you have become reliant upon and which might actually be proving more of a problem than a help, Chapter Six provides some information about a particular therapy within CBT called acceptance therapy which might help you to overcome that.

Mind and body

Often a difficulty in sleeping is not caused by something physical, but by what is going on in the mind. This could be due to a racing, anxious or unhappy mind.

If you have identified that your difficulty might be caused by stress which is leading to your mind racing when you try to sleep, learning more about mindfulness and the techniques of Chapter Two will be helpful. Mindfulness is a tool that can bring you into the present moment when you want to go to sleep, allowing your mind to switch off from its day-to-day challenges and permitting sleep to come naturally.

If the questionnaire helped you to identify that you cannot sleep because negative thoughts keep arising in your mind, or if you have identified that you are feeling worried, anxious or stressed, then turn to Chapters Three to Six, which cover cognitive behavioural therapies and provide visualisation techniques to distract the mind and aid falling sleep.

To get started, the first technique, at the end of this chapter, is a very simple one that can also be taught to children and may be used for any general sleeplessness.

Technique One: The Incoming Tide

Find a comfortable position in which to lie on your
bed, preferably under the covers and with your head
on the pillow. Unless you have some physical difficulty
in doing so, or suffer from sleep apnoea, start by lying
on your back. If you find yourself shifting into another
position during the technique, then it is fine to allow
yourself to do so. Otherwise, try to lie still and not move.
If you have an itch which is annoying you, then move
to scratch it, but apart from that try to remain still.

Imagine that a tide of sleep is coming in
and has just reached your feet.

The tide of sleep is neither hot nor cold. It is the same
temperature as your body. When it touches you, that
part of your body falls asleep. You feel the sensation
of it, tickling a little, as it touches your toes.

Imagine the touch of the sleep, travelling how a rising
tide of water would, rising up from your feet.
Think slowly through the sensation of the sleep reaching
the joints where your toes meet your feet, tickling the
soles of your feet and then reaching your heels.

Feel the sleep creeping around the backs
of your heels, rising up to your ankles and
starting to touch the bottom of your legs.

Next feel the sleep rising like a tide of water would,
putting your legs to sleep a bit at a time. Take care
to feel it at every point – your shins, your knees, your
thighs, perhaps touching the tips of your fingers
if they are by your side. Feel the sleep travelling
up your chest and arms. Don't rush this.

The sleep moves very slowly, sometimes
at a barely noticeable rate.

If you twitch or need to move to satisfy an itch, sometimes
it can feel as if the sleep has retreated. Don't be disturbed
by this – just wait for a moment, re-gather the sensation
of the sleep partway up your body, and then continue
from where you left off. Don't race. Go slowly.

CHAPTER TWO

The Practice of Mindfulness to Aid Sleep

If you struggle to sleep because your mind is racing or turning a problem over when you turn out the lights, mindfulness can be a useful tool to learn. It can help you to clear your mind and relax your body, so that sleep can come naturally.

There is much excitement today around the power of mindfulness. It has become a key part of career development coaching, and is now an accepted practice within mindfulness-based cognitive therapy (or MBCT). Many sleep therapists teach mindfulness as a technique for combatting insomnia, particularly when caused by stress or anxiety.

The principle of mindfulness, in large part, first came to the West through the teachings of Thich Nhat Hanh, a Vietnamese monk who lived in exile in France. His book *The Miracle of Mindfulness* is based upon a letter he wrote in 1974 to the monks within his school of Buddhism back home, giving them advice on how to use mindfulness to endure the persecution they were suffering. It was such a clear explanation of the benefits and techniques of mindfulness practice that when translated into English, it became a classic guide to mindfulness and to the techniques he espoused, based on Buddhist teachings.

Another influential figure in popularising mindfulness in the West was Jon Kabat-Zinn, an American professor of medicine, who founded a Stress Reduction Clinic in the late 1970s. Kabat-Zinn developed a secularised model of mindfulness to be used for managing stress. His method, Mindfulness-Based Stress Reduction (MBSR), introduced mindfulness within a medicalised setting, and became the basis for its adoption within cognitive behavioural therapy.

Mindfulness was originally seen as a technique to clear the mind and switch it into a mode from which it is receptive to meditation and deeper thinking, or as a way to withstand the sufferings of everyday life.

It traces its origins back to ancient China, when mystics used what we now understand as mindfulness techniques to clear their minds in preparation for divination practices. Since then it has formed a key facet of Zen and Buddhist practice for millennia.

In essence, it is the practice of being present in the moment. It involves using one's breath and the repetition of a phrase to calm and clear the mind.

When trying to sleep, if the mind is racing from a busy day and from all the things that must be done or should have been done, it is a powerful tool to quiet your thoughts, either prior to going to bed or once you are in bed and ready for sleep.

It can also be practiced in everyday life when the mind is distracted by anxiety or worry.

In its traditional form, as outlined in the Buddhist *Sutras*, mindfulness is not intended as a way to fall asleep – quite the opposite in fact: it is a practice to be carried out while sitting, as a preparation for meditation. It was and is used by those wishing to meditate – to clear the mind and create a wholesome state under which meditation can begin. The Buddhist meditates on the interdependency and impermanence of all things, and on compassion, as part of his or her journey to awakening.

But as Benson found and first publicised in his book *The Relaxation Response*, mind-clearing and calming techniques such as mindfulness and meditation have a relaxing effect on the body, and a beneficial effect on well-being and health. There have been many studies over the years since that book was published which have demonstrated this link. In 2014, a review of forty-seven independent studies found evidence that meditation reduces anxiety, depression, and pain.[2]

Mindfulness and relaxation techniques are now, for this reason, incorporated into modern 'third-wave' cognitive behavioural therapies, which are used to assist with mental health difficulties and drawn on by sleep therapists to help people with insomnia.

Mindfulness as a tool for enabling sleep

The term 'mindfulness' can be confusing, as it sounds a little bit like your mind should be full. In fact, it means to be aware (mindful) of what is going on around you.

Before trying out mindfulness as a technique for falling asleep, you might want to try the practice during the day, in order to get the hang of it – although it is not difficult.

A Daytime Practice of Mindfulness

Find a comfortable place to sit. You do not need to close your eyes, but you might find it aids your concentration.

Most mindfulness techniques start with the breath. The breath provides an anchor for the thoughts and for the concentration. Breathe slowly in and out, not straining, but being actively conscious of your breath.

It's easy to say 'I don't need a lesson on how to breathe – I do that every day'. The important point is not that you are learning how to breathe or that you should be breathing in some different or special way, but that you are focusing your concentration on your breathing. You are actively controlling it. Remember the sympathetic nervous system discussed in Chapter One, which floods your body with cortisol and adrenaline and speeds up your breathing and your heart rate ready for fight or flight? Well, now you are letting that sympathetic nervous system take a break and consciously taking control of your breathing.

As you breathe in, say a phrase to yourself. Then, as you breathe out, repeat the phrase. By doing so you keep the breaths in and out of regular length over a period of time and give your mind something specific to concentrate on which is tied to the present.

For mindfulness as described in early Buddhist writings, the phrase suggested for use was:

'Experiencing the whole breath, I shall breathe in;
Experiencing the whole breath, I shall breathe out.'

But you can use any phrase. For example:

'I breathe in for one, two, three counts;
I breathe out for one, two, three counts.'

If you find, when trying to relax, that your out-breath is naturally longer than your in-breath, you might want to try:

'I breathe in for one, two counts;
I breathe out for one, two, three counts.'

Or you could simply focus on one phrase for both in and out, such as:

'Rest is an essential part of healing.'

You can use whatever phrase you feel comfortable with – only make sure it is a neutral set of words. It shouldn't be an instruction, any form of nagging or even a pep talk. Try to find a neutral phrase.

While you are thinking about your breath and remembering to say the phrase it is very difficult for your mind to also be trying to solve the problems of the past or the future. You are forced to remain in the present.

To enhance this operation of being in the present, use any or all of your five senses to reflect on what is going on at the present time. What noises can you hear? Is the room warm or cold? If your eyes are open, what colours can you see? Feel the sensation of your body on the chair and the touch of your fingers or hands on your clothes.

If at any time your mind starts to wander or you start to think upsetting thoughts, do not fight the thoughts or try to find arguments against them. Do not follow the thoughts. Accept that they have come into your mind and then let them go. Bring your mind back to your breath. Feel the breath coming into your body, feel it filling up your lungs, and then feel the breath coming out of your body.

It doesn't take long to master the technique of being actively mindful, but try to keep it up for at least ten to fifteen minutes. This allows time for your heart to slow, your natural rate of breathing to slow, and your sympathetic nervous system to take a step back. That's the system that pumps adrenaline into your body so as to make you ready for fight or flight, which was introduced in the last chapter.

You might want to set an alarm to chime when the time you have set for your practice is up. That way you won't be distracted from the present by wondering how much time is left.

Using Mindfulness to Help You Fall Asleep

When using the technique of mindfulness to alleviate sleep difficulties, it is not that the technique cures the mind of its problems or solves them, but that it allows the mind to put them to one side while it concentrates on the task you have given it – for example, that of breathing steadily in and out while repeating a neutral mantra and reflecting on the sensation of your body in the present.

When you turn out the light and close your eyes, it is a time for sleeping, not trying to solve problems. The rest that you get while sleeping will help you cope better with any difficulties you might be facing in your life, so that you can meet them when you are awake and refreshed in the daytime.

You can use the same technique as your daytime practice, but obviously do not set an alarm to chime after fifteen minutes. The technique can also be useful if your sleep is disturbed by waking in the night. As soon as you wake, before you start to become anxious that you will not be able to get back to sleep, and before you start to fret over whether it would be better to remain in bed or rise, use the mindfulness technique to prevent those thoughts taking hold and bring your focus back to your breathing and back to a place from which sleep can return.

Technique Two: A Practice of Mindfulness

Find a comfortable position in which to lie on your bed, preferably under the covers and with your head on the pillow. Unless you have some physical difficulty in doing so, or suffer from sleep apnoea, start by lying on your back, with your hands on your chest. If you find yourself shifting into another position during the technique, then it is fine to allow yourself to do so. Otherwise, try to lie still and not move. If you have an itch which is annoying you, then move to scratch it, but apart from that try to remain still.

Start to think about your breathing and concentrate on it. As you breathe in, your chest rises a little. As you breathe out, your chest falls. Feel the rise and fall of it with your hands on your chest. Don't force your breathing or make it longer than feels natural. Just let it come and go.

As you breathe in, think: 'I'm breathing in, one.'

As you breath out, think: 'I'm breathing out, one, two.'

If your mind starts to fill up with thoughts, do not try to fight or argue against them. Do not follow the thoughts. Accept that they have come into your mind and then let them go.

Bring your mind back to your breath and to the phrase. Feel the breath coming into your body, feel it filling up your lungs, and then feel the breath coming out of your body, your lungs.

Lie still and focus for a moment on your body within the sheets and on the bed. Focus on the feeling of the bedsheets touching your skin.

Next you are going to stop repeating the phrase and instead concentrate on slowly relaxing all the muscles in your body, starting with your forehead. Relax your forehead, then your eyes. Don't rush. Take your time to do it. Relax the muscles in your cheeks and around your mouth. Move down to your chin, your neck, your shoulders. Going slowly and methodically, relax your forearms, chest, stomach, hands, fingers, buttocks, thighs, shins, feet, toes.

While you are doing this, you may find that thoughts keep returning. When they do, let them in. Acknowledge them. Don't analyse them, but let them enter your mind, accept that they are there, and then let them go and empty your mind again by concentrating on your breathing and returning to the progression of relaxing the muscles of your body.

CHAPTER THREE

Dealing with Negative Thoughts When Trying to Sleep

Sometimes sleep can be difficult to achieve because your brain is ticking over with negative thoughts which seem to come from nowhere. They might spark from an initial thought that arose once the light was turned out and which then led to a series of worsening negative thoughts – a downward spiral towards a depressed or sad state of emotion.

Cognitive behavioural therapy focuses on helping people to learn to recognise and interrupt these negative thoughts as soon as they arrive in the mind and to replace them with more appropriate thinking – preventing the negative emotional state taking hold. The techniques taught within CBT can be used at any time of day, but they are also a very useful weapon to have in your armoury when negative thoughts are preventing you from sleeping.

Cognitive behavioural therapy, or CBT, was first developed and popularised in the second half of the twentieth century. It derived from the merging of two types of psychotherapies – behavioural therapies, which developed in the 1950s and 60s and focused on why individuals behave in the way they do, and the cognitive therapies of the psychologist Albert Ellis and the psychiatrist Aaron T. Beck. These cognitive therapists examined how certain ways of thinking can have an impact upon our emotions.

Today, cognitive behavioural therapy is a well-established therapeutic aid for resolving depression and anxiety. It is based on the principle that our thinking processes are influenced by, and in turn influence, our emotions and our behaviours. Hence the merging of the *cognitive* and the *behavioural* therapies.

Identifying and combatting
negative automatic thoughts

Underlying CBT is the principle that somebody's negative thoughts can influence their emotional state, and that a negative emotional state is more likely to give birth to negative thoughts. In this way, a vicious cycle can develop, feeding anxiety or depression, and potentially interfering with an ability to sleep.

Cognitive behavioural therapy calls these negative thoughts 'negative automatic thoughts', or NATs for short.

Examples might be:

'I'm not very clever.'

'I'm so fat.'

'I'm not very likeable.'

'She thinks I'm too shy.'

Here is an example of a series, or downward spiral, of negative automatic thoughts:

'She laughed at me when I made that mistake… She must think I'm stupid… Let's face it, I am stupid… I expect they all think that… Maybe I'll be fired soon… How will I pay the bills?'

Or another example:

'I couldn't fit into those trousers… I'm so fat… No one's going to want to be with me… I think I'm going to stop trying to meet people.'

The key principle of cognitive behavioural therapy is to help the person to spot a negative automatic thought as soon as it arises, and to encourage them to replace the negative thought with a more rational and balanced thought.

Taking the previous examples, both 'She must think I'm stupid' and 'I'm so fat' are negative automatic thoughts. In this particular succession of thoughts, they might be replaced with more rational and balanced ones, such as:

'She laughed at me when I made that mistake. **I guess it was a silly mistake, but actually I very rarely make mistakes, which is probably why she laughed.'**

'I couldn't fit into those trousers. **Although to be fair, I've not been that waist size in years.'**

The key is to RECOGNISE and REPLACE negative automatic thoughts: to recognise a negative automatic thought as soon as it arises, and – particularly if it is likely to lead to a downward spiral of negative thoughts – replace it with a more rational thought.

If you are having difficulty sleeping because you are being assailed by negative thoughts when you turn the light out and close your eyes, then an understanding of these basic principles of cognitive behavioural therapy can go a long way to help you manage these thoughts and find a calmer and quieter frame of mind in which to fall asleep.

Over the next few months, jot down any negative automatic thoughts as they come to you. Recognise them for what they are. You can do this whether the thoughts come during the day or whether they come once you have turned the light off to sleep.

For every negative automatic thought that you write down, beside it write down a more balanced and rational replacement for that thought.

If you find that negative automatic thoughts are arriving when you are in bed trying to sleep, turn on the light for a moment and write down the negative thought. You can either try to replace it at that time with a more rational thought, or you can wait until the morning and do it then. Interrupting and recognising the negative thought is half of the battle. By preparing a more balanced replacement in the morning, you will have it ready for the next time that negative automatic thought occurs to you at night. Only this time you will not need to turn the light on, as you will have your replacement thought already prepared.

At first this might mean that you are interrupting your practice of one of the sleep techniques by turning on the light to write down the negative thought, ready for a replacement to be established, but over time you will build up your reserves of replacement thoughts, allowing you to immediately identify and replace any negative thoughts that arise while you are in bed.

Sometimes when you are anxious about life, it is tempting to give yourself a pep talk or to have an internal argument, with you playing both prosecutor and defender. But this is not conducive to falling asleep. By nature, pep talks and internal dialogues are combative – because of that they stimulate rather than empty your mind, and will work against the sleep techniques.

Going back to Chapter One, when you go to bed and close your eyes to sleep, it is a time for sleep, not for struggle.

Use these two pages to write down negative automatic thoughts that occur to you during the night.

Negative automatic thought

_____

_____

_____

_____

_____

_____

_____

_____

_____

_____

_____

_____

Rational replacement thought

_____

_____

_____

_____

_____

_____

_____

_____

_____

_____

_____

Technique Three: Visualisation A, the Road

Find a comfortable position in which to lie on your bed, preferably under the covers and with your head on the pillow. Unless you have some physical difficulty in doing so, or suffer from sleep apnoea, start by lying on your back. If you find yourself shifting into another position during the technique, then it is fine to allow yourself to do so. Otherwise, try to lie still and not move. If you have an itch which is annoying you, then move to scratch it, but apart from that try to remain still.

If you are being plagued by one or more negative automatic thoughts, turn on the light, write down the negative automatic thought, recognise how it is not balanced, and turn off the light again. Return to the note in the morning and think of a replacement thought that is more balanced and more rational.

Choose a long road that you journey or have journeyed down on a regular basis.

Do not make it a road that you have an emotional attachment to, one which might upset or distract you. Pick a road or journey which is or has been a mundane part of your life at some point.

It might be a road on which you journey to work or college. Or perhaps one you use to take your children to school or to go to the shops. It could be a road you use regularly now, or it might be one near where you have lived in the past. It can be a road in the town or the countryside, so long as there is plenty of detail to remember.

In your mind, walk down that road and try to remember everything that is on your left and on your right as you pass – the houses, the street furniture, the shops, the bus stops, the grass verges.

What colour are the buildings? Do they have any signage? What does that signage say? Are there bins? Bus stops?

What comes first, the launderette or the bakery? What type of material is the pavement or sidewalk made from? Are there streetlamps? If so, what do they look like?

Keep walking slowly down the road towards the end of it, step by step, trying to remember. The intention is not to reach the end of the road, so make sure it is a long one with lots of detail to remember. The intention is to fall asleep during the journey.

CHAPTER FOUR

When Worry or Anxiety Are Keeping You Awake

Worrying is our mind's way of keeping us alert to danger and potential threats, but if we can't turn off worry, or if that worry starts to dominate our thinking, it can go beyond what is useful and instead become destructive to our emotional well-being. Where this happens, worry can lead to obsessive compulsive behaviour (for example a fear of germs leading to constant washing of the hands) or to catastrophising thoughts, meaning imagining worst-case scenarios and dwelling on them.

The last chapter introduced how cognitive behavioural therapy can be used to identify negative thoughts that arise uncalled for in the mind. Cognitive behavioural therapy calls these negative thoughts that arise automatically 'negative automatic thoughts', or NATs for short.

As well as deriving from depression or a negative state of mind, negative automatic thoughts can derive from an underlying state of worry or anxiety. Because these thoughts are not balanced or entirely rational, they contribute to and can worsen your physical feeling of anxiety, leading to a vicious cycle in which anxiety or worry create negative thoughts, and those negative thoughts in turn create worry or anxiety.

An unbalanced or irrational thought could be one which predicts what will happen in the future based upon your fears rather than a knowledge of the facts. Similarly, an unbalanced thought might concentrate on the negative aspects of any situation rather than the neutral or positive ones.

Examples of negative automatic thoughts arising from an underlying anxiety might be:

'If I take that job, I'm likely to fail.'

'They all stopped talking when I came in. I'm sure they were saying they hate me.'

As described in the last chapter, the key is to RECOGNISE and REPLACE negative automatic thoughts arising from worry or anxiety: to recognise the negative automatic thoughts that are posing as normal worries as soon as they arise and replace them with more rational thoughts, particularly if they are likely to lead to a downward spiral.

'Catastrophising' is an extreme version of negative automatic thinking. It is not just unbalanced thinking, but leaping to the worst-case scenario, perhaps even playing it like a video in your mind.

For example, *'She hasn't called. Perhaps she's been involved in a car accident. I can see her terribly hurt.'*

As with negative automatic thoughts, the key is to REC-OGNISE and REPLACE catastrophising thinking before it starts to have a negative impact on your emotional state.

More balanced thinking for the examples given above might include:

'I do have all the qualifications for that job. It's likely I'll be able to do it once I've got used to their systems.'

'They all stopped talking when I came in. I guess the conversation might have just naturally ended at that point, or perhaps they were talking about a friend of mine.'

'She hasn't called. I expect she's busy and forgot.'

Over the next few months, following the instructions in the previous chapter, jot down any negative automatic thoughts related to worry, anxiety or catastrophising thoughts as they come to you. Recognise them for what they are. For every negative automatic thought that you write down, beside it write down a more balanced and rational replacement for that thought.

If you find that the anxiety and worry are overwhelming you, or you recognise that you have developed catastrophising thoughts or some form of compulsive behaviour caused by worry, consider seeking help from a therapist or speaking to your doctor to see if they can arrange some counselling for you. At the back of the book you will find a page with signposts for where you can get more help.

Use these two pages to write down negative automatic thoughts that occur to you during the night.

Negative automatic thought

_____

_____

_____

_____

_____

_____

_____

_____

_____

_____

_____

_____

Rational replacement thought

_____

_____

_____

_____

_____

_____

_____

_____

_____

_____

_____

Technique Four: Visualisation B, the Building

Find a comfortable position in which to lie on your bed, preferably under the covers and with your head on the pillow. Unless you have some physical difficulty in doing so, or suffer from sleep apnoea, start by lying on your back. If you find yourself shifting into another position during the technique, then it is fine to allow yourself to do so. Otherwise, try to lie still and not move. If you have an itch which is annoying you, then move to scratch it, but apart from that try to remain still.

If worries are coming to your mind which you have identified as not entirely balanced, turn on the light and write them down. Turn off the light again, knowing that you will return to the note in the morning, when you will think of a replacement thought that is more balanced. If you already know a more balanced replacement for the worry that you have just had, then replace the negative automatic thought with the more balanced thought, and continue with the sleep technique.

Choose a building that you once knew well. It could be an old school or college that you attended when you were a child, or a library or sports complex in some old town that you used to visit but haven't been to for a long time.

Make sure it isn't a building that creates an emotional reaction in you which is strongly negative or positive.

The building is empty of activity and empty of people.

Starting with the entrance to the grounds of the building, mentally walk towards it. Try to remember what the grounds were like – if there was a playground or yard, were there drawings on the floor? Was there sports equipment in sight? What were the boundaries like – were there railings, a wall or a hedge? What did the building look like from afar; what was it made of?

When you reach the building, enter through the door and try to remember which rooms were in which direction. Try not to associate the building with memories of people, but focus on the rooms themselves, trying to remember what was on the walls, what the floor might have been made of, what the desks or tables and chairs were like. When you have remembered all you can about one room, walk along the corridor to the next, or mentally walk upstairs and think through the rooms there.

Keep walking through the building, going from room to room slowly and methodically, trying to remember. The intention is not to cover the whole of the building, but to fall asleep during the journey through it.

CHAPTER FIVE

Coping with Stress

Stress is defined as a feeling of strain or pressure and it can have many different causes. In the 1960s, two psychiatrists, Thomas Holmes and Richard Rahe, developed a list of forty-three stressful life events, giving each one a score out of 100. The death of a spouse was given the highest score of 100, and divorce was second with a score of 73, followed by marital separation at 65. Other items on the list covered personal injury or illness, difficulties at work, and changes in financial situation, with each holding a score. Holmes and Rahe's research found that a total score of above 300 was likely to put the individual at risk of falling ill, and a score between 150 and 299 would pose a moderate chance of ill health.

Since then studies have consistently shown a link between stress and ill health, with stress causing a higher risk of cardiovascular disease and even making us more susceptible to the common cold.[3]

As described in the first chapter, when our bodies are under pressure the sympathetic nervous system kicks into action, flooding the body with cortisol and adrenaline. When this pressure continues unabated for prolonged periods of time, a condition of stress occurs which can interrupt sleep and leave the body drained and susceptible to ill health.

When you lead a busy life, it can sometimes be difficult to realise how many different things you have to do or are asking your mind to remember. From emails you need to reply to, things you need to buy, people you need to ring, apologies you need to make, visits to friends, relatives or neighbours you need to arrange, cakes that need baking, accounts that need filing... the list can seem endless.

Psychologists differentiate between positive stress and negative stress. Positive stress is what you experience when there is a lot on your plate, but where the things you have to do are providing you with enjoyment and reward. They pose a challenge that you are rising to.

Negative stress is when you might be similarly under pressure, but you feel you are unable to cope. Negative stress can lead to difficulty sleeping and to negative automatic thoughts (see Chapter Three for more details on negative automatic thoughts).

If you have identified that you are under stress and that this is likely to be a cause of your difficulty sleeping, there is work you need to do during the daytime to resolve this. You can use the techniques to get to sleep, but if your body has been in a state of what is known as 'alarm reaction' (i.e. flooded with adrenaline and cortisol) for some time, or if your mind is trying to subconsciously hold a list of a hundred things that need to be done, your sleep is likely to be disturbed.

There is evidence that exercise can help stress: it provides the physical fight or flight reaction that a body flooded with adrenaline has prepared itself for. The exercise produces endorphins and generates physical rather than emotional fatigue, and has been demonstrated to promote better sleep.[4] Research by psychologists Michael Otto and Jasper Smits found that even five minutes of aerobic exercise begins to reduce stress levels and aid well-being, and that exercise sessions do not need to be extensive or regular to be beneficial.

Deciding to walk a few stops rather than take the bus home at the end of a busy day might seem an unattractive prospect, particularly if you are tired, but it will actually promote a better night's sleep, reducing your tiredness the next day and increasing your ability to cope with stress.

In the same way, finding some time during the week to review all the things on your plate can be time well spent. Writing down what needs to be done means that your mind is not having to hold the list during your waking and sleeping hours.

If you are very stressed or busy, finding time outside of what you already have to do can be difficult, but it is well worth doing so. Ideally try to find a regular thirty-minute 'time-out' spot every few weeks and retire to somewhere where you won't be disturbed. Ask those around you not to disturb you for that time, if you are safely able to.

During your time-out session, write down all the things that you need to do, and allocate each one a high, medium or low priority. Base the priorities on realistic timeframes, with the most important to be done first and the least important left for another week, another month, or perhaps even another year.

Then rewrite your list in order of priority, along with possible people who you might be able to ask for help. There is an old saying: 'If you want something done, ask a busy person.' Are you being the busy person who is getting everything done for everyone else? Are there people you can turn to for help instead? Are there people who you have taken work or chores from that you should really tell them to do themselves?

If you are not able to find thirty minutes, then make it just fifteen minutes.

If possible, try to avoid setting this time to be just before you go to bed. Do it earlier in the day.

Keep some paper beside the bed or use the pages at the end of this book to write down any thoughts that occur when you are going to sleep or that wake you in the night, so that they can be added to your list the next time you have a time-out session.

Your time-out session list

Use the space below to write down all the things that are on
your plate at the moment. In the second column, determine
how important they are. In the third column, write down the
names of anyone who might be able to help you with that item.

Item	Priority level (high, medium, low)	Who could help?

Use the pages at the back of this book to re-write the list in order and to write down any ideas or thoughts that arise when you are going to sleep or that wake you in the night.

Technique Five: Visualisation C, the Store

Earlier in the day, take some time out to write down all the things that are on your plate at the moment. Arrange them in order of priority and mark beside them the names of anyone you can think of who might be able to take that item off your plate. Before going to sleep, make sure you have a pen and paper or something you can write on beside the bed.

Find a comfortable position in which to lie on your bed, preferably under the covers and with your head on the pillow. Unless you have some physical difficulty in doing so, or suffer from sleep apnoea, start by lying on your back. If you find yourself shifting into another position during the technique, then it is fine to allow yourself to do so. Otherwise, try to lie still and not move. If you have an itch which is annoying you, then move to scratch it, but apart from that try to remain still.

If, as you are working through the technique, a thought comes to you about something that needs to be done or hasn't been done (or if the thought wakes you when you are sleeping), turn on the light and write it down, then turn off the light again and immediately go back to the sleep technique. In the morning, or at your next time-out session, you will be able to add that thought to your list.

Choose a department store or supermarket which you have visited on enough occasions to be able to vaguely remember what is on the shelves and where.

In your mind, walk into the store and think about what you see immediately. What have staff put around the entrance for you to notice? How many shelves are there? Where are the shelves? What is the floor of the store made of?

Within the store, take the route you would usually take. Think through what is on display on your left and on your right as you progress along the aisles.

If you are in a supermarket, think about what order the produce comes in. Is some of it placed higher or lower? If you are in a department store, what do the display racks look like – are they metal or black? What height are they at?

Progress through the store in a logical order, aisle by aisle. Go slowly and methodically. Don't rush.

The idea is not to reach the checkout tills, but to fall asleep before you get there.

CHAPTER SIX

Sleep Rituals and Worrying About Insomnia

Sometimes, a worry about how much sleep you are getting can become an anxiety in its own right. Chapter Four described how cognitive behavioural therapy recognises that our thoughts can influence our feelings, and that our feelings can influence our thoughts.

You might be having negative automatic thoughts when you go to bed or when you wake in the middle of the night, such as 'I know I'm not going to get any more sleep tonight. I'm going to perform even worse tomorrow.' If so, read or reread Chapter Four and work on finding more rational thoughts to replace this thinking with.

There is a branch of CBT called acceptance and commitment therapy, which was developed by the American clinical psychologist Steven Hayes in the early 1980s. It focuses on helping people to accept the reality of situations and their feelings, and to learn not to overreact to them.

When you can't sleep, an anxiety can take hold about how insomnia will affect your ability to cope in the morning. The traditional advice for this problem was that you should get up rather than toss and turn in bed, but acceptance and commitment therapy suggests that it is better to practise acceptance of your sleep difficulties than to fight against them.

Instead of becoming anxious about your difficulty sleeping, concentrate on a practice of mindfulness, using the repetition of a phrase such as 'Rest is an essential part of healing'. Remind yourself that even if you are not asleep, your body is getting a chance to relax. It is getting an opportunity to process and dispose of the stress hormones that have been flooding your body, allowing your blood pressure to drop, your digestive process to work, and your blood to gently redistribute energy from the digested food to all parts of your body. Accept that you may not get a full eight hours of sleep, but you are likely to get some sleep and your body will get some rest. Identify any overly negative thinking and replace it with more balanced thinking.

Sleep rituals

If you have been suffering from difficulty sleeping for some time, it is possible you have developed a series of actions that you do before you go to bed, and which you feel you must do in order to get a good night's sleep.

These are commonly referred to as sleep rituals, and sometimes they can start to become part of the problem rather than part of the solution.

They include doing things intended to help you wind down before going to bed because you have read or been told that it is good to relax before sleeping – such as taking a bath or having a warm drink.

All of these are definitely good activities for relaxing, and if you are finding that you have a lot of stress or sadness in your life at any time, they are useful for you to do. Extensive research shows that relaxation reduces blood pressure and builds your resistance to stress-related diseases.

But if these activities have become things that *must* be done before you feel you can sleep, then that belief can be counted as an obsessive thought to be identified and replaced with more rational thinking, as with any other negative automatic thought.

Some people can fall asleep on noisy tube trains or aeroplanes in the middle of the day. Small children can fall asleep in their seat with a party going on at full blast around them. While it's good to mitigate the environmental factors that might be contributing to you dropping off, and to do things to calm your body after a stressful day, don't let these things become obsessive.

If you think you feel anxious about sleeping when you haven't been able to carry out your sleep rituals, try dropping one of these rituals and using the practices of cognitive behavioural therapy outlined in Chapters Three and Four to alleviate your anxiety. Work towards finding more rational thoughts to replace a fear that you will not be able to sleep because a sleep ritual has not been completed.

Technique Six: Down the Rabbit Hole

Find a comfortable position in which to lie on your bed, preferably under the covers and with your head on the pillow. Unless you have some physical difficulty in doing so, or suffer from sleep apnoea, start by lying on your back. If you find yourself shifting into another position during the technique, then it is fine to allow yourself to do so. Otherwise, try to lie still and not move. If you have an itch which is annoying you, then move to scratch it, but apart from that try to remain still.

Slow your breathing in and out to a steady pace. Concentrate on your breathing for a few minutes. As you breathe in, say in your mind, 'Rest is an essential part of healing.' As you breathe out, repeat the phrase. Don't try to force your breath to be faster or slower than comes naturally to you.

Imagine that you are sitting in an open field with your back to a tree, and you see that there is a neat and fairly wide hole in the grass a few yards in front of you.

You decide to go and investigate the hole. You find that you are able to climb into it and down the walls of the hole. They support you. It is neither too hot nor too cold in the hole; it is just the right temperature.

It is not dirty or muddy and there are grips for your hands. The walls support your feet and allow you to climb down. You do not have any fear of falling.

As you climb down you look up at the circle of daylight above your head: it gets smaller and smaller as you descend. Below you is another circle of light, also very small.

You keep climbing until the hole above your head is just a small pinprick.

CHAPTER SEVEN

Should I Be Meditating?

When you are not sure what it is all about, meditation can seem a little mysterious or curious. What are people actually doing when they are meditating? Is a practice of mindfulness the same as meditation? Is your mind supposed to be blank or full of thought when you meditate?

This chapter aims to provide a brief introduction to meditation, to demystify it, and to allow you to decide whether it is something you would like to look into further or try.

Essentially, the word 'meditate', according to the Oxford English Dictionary, means 'focus one's mind for a period of time' and/or 'think deeply about (something)'. If you have got the hang of mindfulness, you will see that meditation is therefore significantly different. When practising mindfulness, the idea is to clear your mind of thought by concentrating on your breath and a repeated phrase, and to be present in the moment. By contrast, meditation is a *thinking* or *contemplative* practice.

Mindfulness and meditation within Buddhism

Like mindfulness, the formal practice of meditation has its origins millennia ago in the East. In its traditional form, it is one of a set of Buddhist practices that together make up the 'Noble Eightfold Path'. Buddhists believe that following this path can eventually lead to insight into the true nature of reality.

The practices of mindfulness and meditation are two separate parts or spokes of the Noble Eightfold Path (which is often visualised as a wheel), called 'Right Effort' and 'Right Concentration' respectively.

Under Right Effort, the follower of the Noble Eightfold Path works to generate a wholesome state under which his or her enlightenment can be achieved. Mindfulness (or *sati*) is used for clearing or 'purifying' the mind and for the overcoming of sorrow. It is used as a preparation for meditation.

Under Right Concentration, the follower uses meditation (or *samadhi*) to contemplate upon a number of prescribed subjects. These include interdependency (a belief held by some Buddhists that we are all connected and are one and the same), compassion (practising seeing through the eyes of others), and impermanency (which involves meditating on death and the cycle of life).

Buddhists interpret these ancient teachings in various ways, with some incorporating them into their lives to a greater or lesser extent. In Thailand, for example, many young men take a break from their everyday lives at some point to become a monk, living an ascetic life and attempting to turn away from material desires. This might be for a year or just a few months. Meanwhile, many modern Buddhists find ways to incorporate a practice of meditation into busy daily lives.

Bringing mindfulness and meditation into our lives

It was really only in the late twentieth century that the Western world began to consider and accept the benefits that mindfulness and meditation can bring, and to find ways to bring these practices into its own philosophies and thinking.

Nowadays, 'mindfulness' is the current buzzword. It's unlikely you will go on a personal development course at work without it being raised in one form or another. It has spawned an empire of self-help manuals, of games, cards, notebooks, and more – constant reminders of how and when to be mindful. And with the interest in mindfulness has come a renewed curiosity about meditation.

If you would like to meditate, it does not need to be anything more complicated than sitting quietly and thinking through a problem that you would like to work through.

The 'time-out' session of the previous chapter is a form of meditation, in that you are taking some time to sit in a quiet place, perhaps after a few minutes of mind-clearing mindfulness, to think through your list of things to be done or arranged.

If you can find time in your day or week to spend a few minutes practising mindfulness, followed by a few minutes of meditating on plans or problems, both your body and mind will benefit, facilitating better sleep when you go to bed.

Using meditation time to think through events of the past that are upsetting can have a negative effect on your emotional well-being and therefore on your ability to sleep. If you think there are things from your past that you want to explore, it is best to do so within a therapy session, where there is a therapist at hand to help and guide you. At the end of the book, there are details about where to go to get more help or to find a therapist.

Technique Seven: A Second Mindfulness Practice

Find a comfortable position in which to lie on your bed, preferably under the covers and with your head on the pillow. Unless you have some physical difficulty in doing so, or suffer from sleep apnoea, start by lying on your back. If you find yourself shifting into another position during the technique, then it is fine to allow yourself to do so. Otherwise, try to lie still and not move. If you have an itch which is annoying you, then move to scratch it, but apart from that try to remain still.

Slow your breathing in and out to a steady pace. Concentrate on your breathing for a few minutes.

Feel the sensation of the sheets touching you, of your head on the pillow, of your legs and feet on the bed.

Start to use your senses to think about what you can hear. Is there noise in the room, or outside the room? Is there the sound of any neighbours, or the sound of wind or rain outside the window?

What is the temperature in your room? Are you hot or cold? Warm or cool?

Think about the room, think about the things in
the room, think about the walls of the room.

Then bring your consciousness to what is outside your
room – to the other rooms in your home, to the loft
space or apartment above, to the roof of your building.
Imagine you are passing up through them.

Don't rush. Take your time.

Think about the wider sphere outside your building, the
grounds that it is in, the garden or gardens, a park or car park
perhaps. Think about the area outside your house or apartment, your street. Is it windy? Where is the wind blowing
from or to? Imagine you are there looking at the things below
you, studying them. You are not cold. You are perfectly warm.

Imagine you are lifting up until you are far above your
town, village or city, in the air. Lift up until you are at the
dark edge of space. There is a line attaching you to your
bed. You can use it at any time to return. You fly out a
little further until you start to see the stars around you.

Take your time with this technique. The aim is not to
reach the moon, but to fall asleep on the journey.

CHAPTER EIGHT

Putting It All Together

Getting a good night's sleep is as much about figuring out why you are not sleeping and finding techniques to mitigate the impact of those issues on your ability to fall asleep as it is about finding a *way* to fall asleep.

This book has provided eight techniques that you can use when you have turned off the light and wish to go to sleep, but all the activities below – which form a summary of all the guidance in this book – if carried out on a regular basis will help get your mind and body better prepared to fall asleep in a timely fashion and to keep asleep.

During your daytime

1. Make space in your life, at least every few weeks, for a period of 'time-out' in a calm and quiet place where you won't be disturbed. Try to make the time-out session at least fifteen minutes, and preferably twenty or thirty minutes.

    Use the first few minutes of the time to practise mindfulness, concentrating on your breath and on a phrase which will bring your mind to the present. This allows your body to relax and your sympathetic nervous system to take a step back.

    Use the rest of the session to contemplate any problems you are currently facing. Or use the time to list everything on your plate, to arrange the list into high, medium and low priorities, and to think of people who can help you or who you could delegate tasks to.

2. Make space in your week for exercise, even if it is only briskly walking a few stops rather than catching the bus, or walking upstairs rather than taking the lift. Even ten

or fifteen minutes of exercise on a periodic basis will be beneficial, but do more if you have the time and are able. Invest in a pedometer if you think that will help to remind you to build exercise into your life.

3. The practice of mindfulness can be carried out at any time and is beneficial because it helps promote relaxation. But there are many other things we can do to help us live in the present and concentrate on something other than our worries, such as dancing, singing along to the radio, practising yoga, exercising, enjoying nature, walking in a new town or city, or meeting up with friends. Try and find a way to make one or two things of this sort part of your everyday life.

4. If you find you are disturbed by anxious thoughts which are overly negative, or by catastrophising (where you are jumping to the worst-case scenario), write these thoughts down. These are called negative automatic thoughts. Reflect on how and in what way these thoughts might not be entirely rational or based on the true facts of the situation, and think of more balanced thoughts that can

replace them. Write down the replacement thoughts so that if you have a negative automatic thought when you are trying to sleep, you will have a replacement for it immediately to hand.

If you are feeling overwhelmed by sadness, stress, anxiety or worry, consider speaking to your doctor or a therapist. There are details at the back of the book regarding where you can turn to for help.

For your sleeping time

1. If your room is overly light or noisy, invest in an eye mask and/or earplugs.

2. If you know you have a problem with night sweats and hot flushes, switch your bedding for a light sheet covered by a duvet, eiderdown or other heavier bedding which can be quickly thrown off.

3. If you're so hot when you go to bed that you cannot sleep, step into a cold shower for one to two seconds, before putting some light cotton underwear on while you are still damp and getting back into bed.

4. Ensure you have some writing materials by your bed in case thoughts wake you in the night.

5. If you are disturbed by a negative automatic thought when you turn off the light, or if one wakes you in the night, think of a more balanced replacement thought. If you do not have one prepared, identify and write down the thought, and in the morning consider a more balanced replacement. Write that replacement thought down so that it is ready for next time.

6. If you are disturbed by a sudden thought of something that must be done when you turn off the light, or if such a thought wakes you in the night, write it down and try to immediately return to sleep or to a sleep technique. In the morning, you can add this to the list you keep during your time-out sessions.

7. Work through a sleep technique slowly, methodically, and calmly.

8. If you wake in the night, combat anxiety with an understanding that you are getting rest simply by being in bed and getting a little sleep.

At all times, bear in mind that difficulty sleeping is something that affects most people at some point in their life. Sleeplessness can arise for a multitude of reasons, as covered in the chapters of this book, but if you are in bed, lying down, and relaxing, your body is getting a chance to rest.

You may not be able to change your situation if you are facing difficulties in your life, but getting a good night's sleep will help you cope better with life's challenges. Eliminating environmental and physical factors that are preventing you sleeping, finding space for your time-out sessions, and gaining a brief understanding of CBT, mindfulness or meditation can all be worthwhile, helping you to sleep better, cope better and move towards a place of better well-being.

Technique Eight: The Flying Bed

Find a comfortable position in which to lie on your bed, preferably under the covers and with your head on the pillow. Unless you have some physical difficulty in doing so, or suffer from sleep apnoea, start by lying on your back. If you find yourself shifting into another position during the technique, then it is fine to allow yourself to do so. Otherwise, try to lie still and not move. If you have an itch which is annoying you, then move to scratch it, but apart from that try to remain still.

Slow your breathing in and out to a steady pace.
Concentrate on your breath for a few minutes.

Concentrate on slowly relaxing all the muscles in your body, starting with your forehead. Relax your forehead, then your eyes. Don't rush. Take your time to do it. Relax the muscles in your cheeks and around your mouth. Move down to your chin, your neck, your shoulders. Going slowly and methodically, relax your forearms, chest, stomach, hands, fingers, buttocks, thighs, shins, feet, toes.

Feel the sensation of the sheets touching you, of your head on the pillow, of your legs and feet on the bed.

Imagine that your bed has lifted up and is carrying you through the window and out into the dark night.

Feel it floating there. It is a bit like a flying carpet in a children's story. The sheets flap a little in a light breeze.

It is neither too cold nor too hot and the weather cannot touch you. You do not sit up; you lie still. If it is raining or snowing, the rain or snow falls to either side of the bed.

You can feel the bed gently moving. It is a pleasant feeling. The bed flies out over your neighbour-hood in a straight line over the buildings, parks or fields. Think of what it passes over.

It doesn't take a route you would follow in a car. Try and imagine what it would fly over, which houses or apartments or parks or lanes or roads it would cross.

Take your time. Don't rush.

The idea is not to reach the next town, but to fall asleep on the journey there.

Where to Find Further Help and Information

UK

You may be able to access a cognitive behavioural therapist through the NHS by contacting your GP, who will be able to advise you on how to find and access local services.

Or you can apply directly to the NHS Improving Access to Psychological Therapies (IAPT) service. You can find your local service on the website: www.nhs.uk/service-search/.

If you would prefer to see a private therapist (which might be quicker to arrange, but they will usually charge for appointments), then the British Association for Counselling and Psychotherapy (BACP) holds a directory of registered

and non-registered therapists at www.bacp.co.uk/ and the British Association for Behavioural and Cognitive Psychotherapists (BABCP) holds a register of accredited CBT therapists at
www.cbtregisteruk.com/.

The organisation Mind also has lots of information about how and where to find a therapist who is right for you. Its website is:
www.mind.org.uk/.

USA and Canada

The Association for Behavioural and Cognitive Therapies (ABCT) has information about therapists in the USA and Canada and a directory to find a therapist close to you on its website:
www.abct.org.

Australia

If you would like to receive help from a CBT therapist, contact your GP and ask for a referral. If you are at school or university, your counsellor may also be able to refer you to a CBT therapist.

The following websites also provide directories of psychologists and clinical psychologists who may offer CBT therapy:

www.psychology.org.au/Find-a-Psychologist
www.acpa.org.au/find-a-clinical-psychologist/

MY SLEEP NOTES

References

[1]Collaborative Group on Hormonal Factors in Breast Cancer, 'Type and timing of menopausal hormone therapy and breast cancer risk: individual participant meta-analysis of the worldwide epidemiological evidence', The Lancet, vol. 394, no. 10204, 29 August 2019, pp. 1159–68, doi:10.1016/S0140-6736(19)31709-X.

[2]M. Goyal, S. Singh, E. M. Sibinga et al., 'Meditation programs for psychological stress and well-being: a systematic review and meta-analysis', JAMA Internal Medicine, vol. 174, no. 3, March 2014, pp. 357–68, doi:10.1001/jamainternmed.2013.13018.

[3]S. Cohen, W. J. Doyle, D. P. Skoner et al., 'Social Ties and Susceptibility to the Common Cold', JAMA: The Journal of the American Medical Association, vol. 277, no. 24, 25 June 1997, pp. 1940–4, doi:10.1001/jama.1997.03540480040036. See also W. J. Edmunds, G. F. Medley, and C. J. O'Callaghan, letter in response to 'Social Ties and Susceptibility to the Common Cold', JAMA: The Journal of the American Medical Association, vol. 278, no. 15, 1997, DOI: 10.1001/jama.1997.03550150035018.

[4]M. W. Otto and J. A. J. Smits, Exercise for Mood and Anxiety: Proven Strategies for Overcoming Depression and Enhancing Well-Being, Oxford University Press, 2011.

Further Reading

The Miracle of Mindfulness: The Classic Guide to Meditation by the World's Most Revered Master, Thich Nhat Hanh (1975)

Full Catastrophe Living: How to Cope with Stress, Pain and Illness Using Mindfulness Meditation, Jon Kabat-Zinn (1990)

The Relaxation Response, Herbert Benson, M.D. (1975)

Buddha's Brain: The Practical Neuroscience of Happiness, Love and Wisdom, Rick Hanson, PhD with Richard Mendius, M.D. (2009)

Exercise for Mood and Anxiety: Proven Strategies for Overcoming Depression and Enhancing Well-Being, Michael W. Otto, PhD, and Jasper A. J. Smits, PhD (2011)

Retrain Your Brain: Cognitive Behavioral Therapy in 7 Weeks: A Workbook for Managing Depression and Anxiety, Seth J. Gillihan, PhD (2016)